Diets and Lifestyles of the Worlds Oldest Peoples

Thousands of books are written on diets. But not many if any on how the longest lived communities in the world live and what they actually eat.

This book is a study of the lifestyles and diets of the four longest lived communities in the world. All of these locations have a higher proportion of centenarians and super centenarians per hundred thousand of population as well as many persons who live to their 130s-140s and even older.

The longevity communities in this book are:

I0412542

- Okinawa, Japan

- The Republic of Abkhazia next to southern Russia.

- Vilcabamba, Ecuador

- Hunza People of northern Pakistan

Lots of information is also provided about the lifestyles of these localities and other longevity factors are elaborated on too.

We also provide some Diet and Lifestyle steps to get you started on losing weight and improving your health starting today.

Come join us as we learn more about how we should live and eat to optimize long term health through the best Lifestyles and Diets !

Diets and Lifestyles of the Worlds Oldest Peoples

Diets and Lifestyles of the Worlds Oldest
Peoples

Diets and Lifestyles of the Worlds Oldest Peoples

MEDICAL & GENERAL DISCLAIMER

(Have to do this for the Lawyers)

This disclaimer is to clarify my role as Author of this book and to provide some legal protection:

- The Author is not a medical professional so any claims he makes are not backed up by any type of professionally accepted scientific evidence or formal training on his part.

- The Author is not a certified nutritionist and makes not claims about the diets suggested.

- The Author does not make any claims to cure any medical conditions or to guarantee any increases in individual lifespans

- The Author is not an herbalist or pharmacologist so is not claiming that his suggestions in using herbs are based on any specialized expertise on his part. Caution and review of suggested supplements with experts is always recommended to make sure the individual doesn't have any medical side effects.

- The Author is not a Minister or Priest in any formal religious tradition so does not claim any special expert knowledge in those traditions.

- Any information or pictures in this book which the Author did not write or create may have been copied and modified from publicly available sources on the internet

Diets and Lifestyles of the Worlds Oldest Peoples

Diets and Lifestyles of the Worlds Oldest Peoples

Other books by Martin K. Ettington

Spiritual and Metaphysics Books:
Prophecy: A History and How to Guide
God Like Powers and Abilities
Enlightenment for Newbies
Removing Illusions to Find True
        Happiness
Using the Scientific Method to Study
        the Paranormal
A Compendium of Metaphysics and
        How to Guides (Six books
        together in one volume)
Love from the Heart
The Enlightenment Experience
Learn Your Soul's Purpose
Pursuing Enlightenment
A Modern Man's Search for Truth
Use Intuition and Prophecy to
        Improve Your Life
The Handbook of Spiritual and Energy
        Healing

Longevity & Immortality:
Physical Immortality: A History and
        How to Guide
The Commentaries of Living Immortals
Records of Extremely Long Lived
        Persons
Enlightenment and Immortality
Longevity Improvements from Science
The 10 Principles of Personal
        Longevity
Telomeres & Longevity
The Diets and Lifestyles of the Worlds
        Oldest Peoples
The Longevity Six Books Bundle

Science Fiction:
Out of This Universe
Personal Freedom-Parts 1 & 2
The Psychic Soldier Series:
    Book 1-Himalayan Journey

Book 2-A Soldier is Born
Book 3-Fighting For Right
Book 4-Earth Protector
The Immortality Sci Fi Bundle

The God Like Powers Series:
Human Invisibility
Invulnerability and Shielding
Teleportation
Psychokinesis
Our Energy Body, Auras, and
Thoughtforms

The God Like Powers Series—
        Volume 1 Compilation
The Yoga Discovery Series:
Yoga-An Ancient Art Form
Hatha Yoga-Helping you Live Better
Raja Yoga-Through the Ages
The Yoga Discovery Package

Business & Coaching Books:
Creating, Publishing, & Marketing
        Practitioner Ebooks
Building a Successful Longevity
        Coaching Business
Why Become a Coach?
The Professional Coaching Success
Trilogy
2020-Make Money Writing and Selling
        Books
The 2020 Handbook of High Paying
        Work Without a College Degree

Science, Technology, and Misc.
Future Predictions By and Engineer &
        Seer
The Unusual Science & Technology
        Bundle
The Real Atlantis-In the Eye of the
        Sahara

Diets and Lifestyles of the Worlds Oldest Peoples

Are Cryptozoological Animals Real or Imaginary?

Real Time Travel Stories From a Psychic Engineer

Removing Limits On Our Consciousness-And Thinking Outside the Box

33 Incredible True Survival Stories

How to Survive Anything: From the Wilderness to Man Made Disasters

All About Mars Journeys and Settlement

Mining the Asteroid Belt

Ancient History

The Real Atlantis-In the Eye of the Sahara

Ancient & Prehistoric Civilizations

Ancient & Prehistoric Civilizations-Book Two

The History of Antediluvian Giants

The Antediluvian History of Earth

Ancient Underground Cities and Tunnels

Strange Objects Which Should Not Exist

Strange and Ancient Places in the USA

A Theory of Ancient Prehistory And Giant Aliens

Aliens and Space

Aliens and Secret Technology

Aliens Are Already Among Us

Designing and Building Space Colonies

Humanity and the Universe

All About Moon Bases

All About Mars Journeys and Settlement

The Space and Aliens Six Books Bundle

A Theory of Ancient Prehistory and Giant Aliens

The Space Colonies and Space Structures Coloring Book

All About Asteroids

The Longevity Training Series

(A transcription of the online Multimedia Longevity Coaching Training Program)
The Personal Longevity Training Series-Book1-Long Lived Persons
The Personal Longevity Training Series-Book2-Your Soul's Purpose
The Personal Longevity Training Series-Book3-Enable Your Life Urge
The Personal Longevity Training Series-Book4-Your Spiritual Connection
The Personal Longevity Training Series-Book5-Having Love in Your Heart
The Personal Longevity Training Series-Book6-Energy Body Health
The Personal Longevity Training Series-Book7-The Science of Longevity
The Personal Longevity Training Series-Book8-Physical Body Health
The Personal Longevity Training Series-Book9-Avoiding Accidents
The Personal Longevity Training Series-Book10-Implementing These Principles

The Personal Longevity Training Series-Books One Thru Ten

These books are all available in digital and printed formats from my website and on Amazon, Barnes & Noble, Apple ITunes, and many other sites

My Books Website is: http://mkettingtonbooks.com

Diets and Lifestyles of the Worlds Oldest Peoples

See our website at http://mkettingtonbooks.com

If you have any questions about this book or other subjects please contact the Author at:

mke@mkettingtonbooks.com

Diets and Lifestyles of the Worlds Oldest Peoples

Diets and Lifestyles of the Worlds Oldest Peoples

Table of Contents

Diets and Lifestyles of the Worlds Oldest Peoples

Diets and Lifestyles of the Worlds Oldest Peoples

We struggle with eating healthily, obesity, and access to good nutrition for everyone. But we have a great opportunity to get on the right side of this battle by beginning to think differently about the way that we eat and the way that we approach food-Marcus Samuelsson

Introduction

Since becoming immersed in the subject of Longevity and Physical Immortality for the last seven years, I've spent most of my time focusing on the non physical aspects of our health and longevity.

What I've learned about long term health is embodied the "10 Principles of Personal Longevity" which is discussed briefly later in this book.

However, the biggest immediate problem which most people suffer in the United States today is being overweight, obese, too fat-- whatever you want to call it.

This condition of being overweight affects the entire population and is only getting worse as the chart below shows:

Overweight and obesity

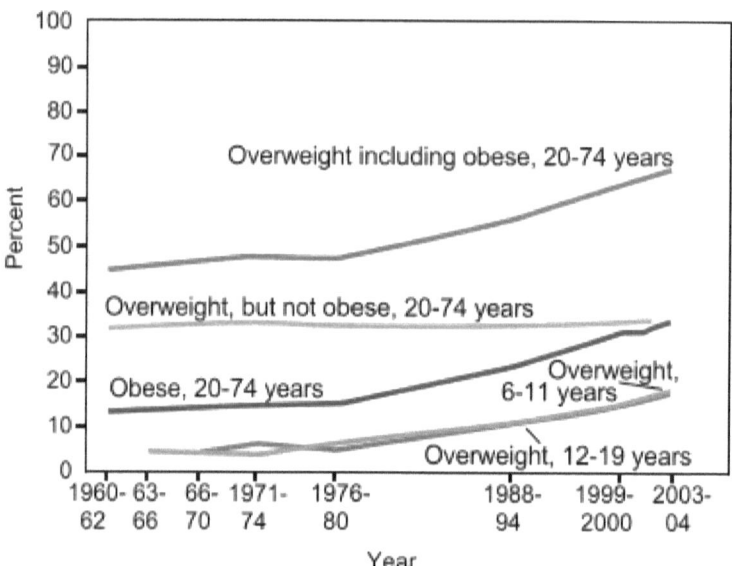

SOURCES: Centers for Disease Control and Prevention, National Center for Health Statistics, Health, United States, 2006, Figure 13. Data from National Health and Nutrition Examination Survey

You probably also know that obesity is one of the prime causes of many chronic diseases including: Diabetes, Heart Disease, High Blood Pressure, and much more.

Most people want to solve their weight problems first before looking at improving their long term health and longevity--and this makes obvious sense.

There are thousands of diet books and diet centers out there--so I wondered for a long time--What unique contribution can I make?

It came to me in an epiphany--That I've developed the correct long term health principles and longevity principles--but most people will not learn the 10 Principles of Personal Longevity in a serious way until they can see a path towards ending their weight and obesity problems.

Diets and Lifestyles of the Worlds Oldest Peoples

The solution is to take what I know about the world's longest lived cultures and teach people more about what they eat and how they live.

These are real world examples--so why not use them?

Therefore, I've been learning a lot more about these long lived communities and this book is a presentation about those communities lifestyles and what they eat.

I've also included comparison matrixes and summaries of what I learned they all have in common.

Finally, a diet and lifestyle program is recommended for those willing to follow thee examples.

I strongly recommend that you don't make any major diet or lifestyle changes according to this book unless you have consulted your Doctor and/or additional certified Diet and Nutrition Professionals.

Hope you enjoy the book and it leads you to our full Longevity training program on the 10 Principles.

Diets and Lifestyles of the Worlds Oldest Peoples

Diets and Lifestyles of the Worlds Oldest Peoples

The Worlds Longest Lived Communities

I've avoided the subject of the best longevity diets for years since there are thousands of diets out there and I didn't feel I had anything new to present on the subject.

However, I recently spent more time reading about the lifestyles of very long lived persons and decided that the examples they and their communities represent needed to be shown to the world.

There have been many previous researchers and writers on the subject on healthily diets, but I thought my perspective on longevity might be unique since I focus mainly on successful lifestyles....and diet is part of the lifestyle.

The first thing I did in my research was to narrow down choices for the longest lived communities featured in this book

My criteria for picking long lived communities were several:

- An unusually high proportion of the population is over one hundred years

- The community has a well defined culture

- Sufficient population so that lifestyles and eating habits are a common "Standard" model

- Fairly isolated communities which haven't been too "contaminated" by Western Cultures

The result was a decision to focus on these four communities around the world:

- Okinawa, Japan- This island has a very healthy lifestyle and has been extensively studied for their longevity. Estimate 1.3 million population 2015.

- The Republic of Abkhazia next to southern Russia. Population of 243,000 in 2012 census. A 1970 census had established Abkhazia, then an autonomous region within Soviet Georgia, as the longevity capital of the world. Very many persons over 100 years of age and even into 120-130 age range.

- Vilcabamba, Ecuador-This small community in the mountains of Ecuador is also known as "The Valley of Longevity" . Population around 7,000 persons and a very high proportion of persons living to 130-140 years old

- The Hunza People of Pakistan-In far northern Pakistan at an elevation of 8,200 feet have many people over one hundred and persons who are 130-150 years old. An estimated population of 60,000

****

In the next Chapter we will review the Okinawa lifestyle.....

Diets and Lifestyles of the Worlds Oldest Peoples

Okinawa Lifestyle

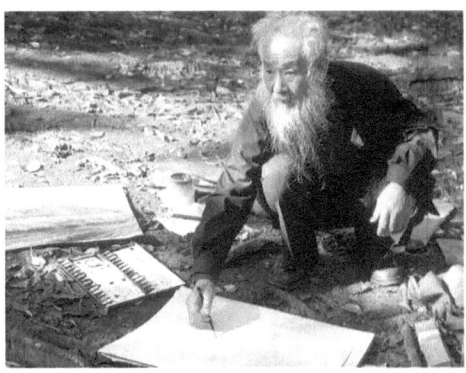

Okinawans have great respect for each other and the elderly:

• One most prominent custom on Okinawa is bowing. Bowing is an Okinawan greeting...having the same meaning as shaking hands in America. It also shows respect. The deeper the bow, the greater the respect. Normally, one would not bow deeply to a shopkeeper when making a purchase...nor would it be acceptable to merely nod to a person of honor. You will find that Okinawans do not often shake hands. If in doubt, by all means bow.

• Other Okinawan customs deal with matters of courtesy. First, show respect for the elderly, as they have an exalted place in Okinawan society. Second, you should not walk into Japanese homes, shrines or temples wearing shoes. If you see a tatami (grass) mat, it is usually a clue to take your shoes off. When in doubt, observe our hosts and do as they do. Generally, you do not have to leave a tip at restaurants, hotels, bars or in taxicabs.

Extract of an article from theguardian.com (Wilson, 2001)

So what are the Okinawans doing right? The simple answer is, of course, that they are living a depressingly healthy lifestyle. They don't get drunk every night. They don't eat loads of fast-food and they don't get really, really stressed out over work. They do not chain smoke or work closely with asbestos. Nor do they indulge in class A drugs, a couch-potato lifestyle and the belief that swallowing their anger/grief/fear/panic, packing it all down and screwing the lid on tight is a good way to deal with the bad times. Oh, and they don't live all alone in their old age in 25-storey blocks of flats with a half-dead cat and no visitors from one day to the next.

No - as you may have guessed, the Okinawans (at least the older ones, who've not yet been tainted by western society) are regular paragons of clean, healthy, spiritually-sound living. They eat well, they eat little, they're surrounded by lots of loving family members and they're well into their martial arts and meditation.

What makes their prescription for longevity interesting, however, is in the detail. For a start, the soya. These people eat a lot of soya, and it clearly does them no harm whatsoever, even if it's not keeping them alive. Then there's all the carbohydrate - they get about two thirds of their calories from it. So forget about Hollywood's high-protein, low-carb "zone" diet and those half-baked theories that we're hunter gatherers and poorly suited to eating the fruits of agriculture: you finish your sandwich, love. Some other tips from Okinawa: eat up your sweet potatoes and your watermelon (surely a completely useless fruit?). The Okinawans, who speak a language similar to ancient Japanese, can't get enough of them.

****

We will discuss Okinawan's diet more in the next chapter

Diets and Lifestyles of the Worlds Oldest Peoples

Okinawa Diet

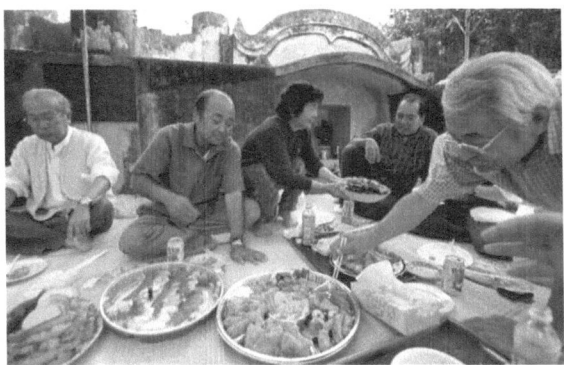

People from the Ryukyu Islands (of which Okinawa is the largest) have a life expectancy among the highest in the world, although the male life expectancy rank among Japanese prefectures has plummeted in recent years.

The traditional diet of the islanders contains 30% green and yellow vegetables. Although the traditional Japanese diet usually includes large quantities of rice, the traditional Okinawa diet consists of smaller quantities of rice; instead the staple is the purple-fleshed Okinawan sweet potato. The Okinawan diet has only 30% of the sugar and 15% of the grains of the average Japanese dietary intake.

The traditional diet also includes a tiny amount of fish (less than half a serving per day) and more in the way of soy and other legumes (6% of total caloric intake). Pork is highly valued, and every part of the pig is eaten, including internal organs. However, pork is primarily only eaten at monthly festivals and the daily diet is almost entirely plant based

Between a sample from Okinawa where life expectancies at birth and 65 were the longest in Japan, and a sample from Akita Prefecture where the life expectancies were much shorter, intakes of calcium, Iron and vitamins A, B1, B2, C, and the proportion of energy from proteins and fats were significantly higher in Okinawa than in Akita. And intakes of carbohydrates and salt were lower in Okinawa than in Akita.

The quantity of pork consumption per person a year in Okinawa is larger than that of the Japanese national average. For example, the quantity of pork consumption per person a year in Okinawa in 1979 was 7.9 kg (17 lb) which exceeded by about 50% that of the Japanese national average.

The dietary intake of Okinawans compared to other Japanese circa 1950 shows that Okinawans consumed:

- fewer total calories (1785 vs 2068)

- less polyunsaturated fat (4.8% of calories vs. 8%)

- less rice (154 grams vs 328g)

- significantly less wheat, barley and other grains (38 g vs. 153g)

- less sugars (3g vs. 8g)

- more legumes (71g vs 55g)

- significantly less fish (15g vs 62g)

- significantly less meat and poultry (3g vs 11g)

- less eggs (1g vs 7 g)

- less dairy (<1g vs 8 g)

- much more sweet potatoes (849g vs 66g)

- less other potatoes (2g vs 47)

- less fruit (<1g vs 44g)

- no pickled vegetables (0g vs 42)

In short, the Okinawans circa 1950 ate sweet potatoes for 849 grams of the 1262 grams of food that they consumed, which constituted 69% of their total calories.

Diets and Lifestyles of the Worlds Oldest Peoples

An Okinawan reaching 100 years of age has typically had a diet consistently averaging about one calorie per gram of food and has a BMI of 20.4 in early adulthood and middle age·

****

Next we move to Abkhazia next to Southern Russia to learn about who they are and their lifestyle

Diets and Lifestyles of the Worlds Oldest Peoples

Diets and Lifestyles of the Worlds Oldest Peoples

Abkhazia Lifestyle

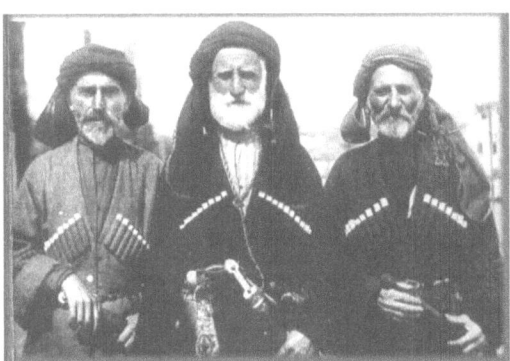

Most of the information about the lifestyle of Abkasian people is taken from the article Abkhazia: Ancients of the Caucasus, by John Robbins (Robbins)

 "Certainly no area in the world," Leaf wrote, "has the reputation for long-lived people to match that of the Caucasus in southern Russia." And in all the Caucasus, the area most renowned for its extraordinary number of healthy centenarians (people above the age of 100) was Abkhazia (pronounced "ab-KAY-zha"). A 1970 census had established Abkhazia, then an autonomous region within Soviet Georgia, as the longevity capital of the world. "We were eager to see the centenarians," Leaf said, "and Abkhazia seemed to be the place to do so."

Abkhazia covers three thousand square miles between the eastern shores of the Black Sea and the crestline of the main Caucasus range. It is bordered on the north by Russia, and on the south by Georgia.

Diets and Lifestyles of the Worlds Oldest Peoples

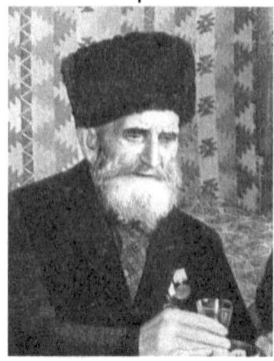

Shirali Mislimov at 168 years old

Prior to Dr. Leaf's visit, claims had been widely circulated for life spans reaching 150 years among the Abkhazians. Just a few years earlier, Life magazine had run an article with photos of Shirali Muslimov, said to be 161 years old. In one of the photos, Muslimov was shown with his third wife. He told the reporter that he had married her when he was 110, that his parents had both lived to be over 100, and that his brother had died at the age of 134.

Muslimov had passed away by the time of Leaf's studies. But a woman named Khfaf Lasuria had also been featured in the Life article. Leaf wanted to meet her, and he found her in the Abkhasian village of Kutol, where she sang in a choir made up entirely, he was told, of Abkhazian centenarians.

Diets and Lifestyles of the Worlds Oldest Peoples

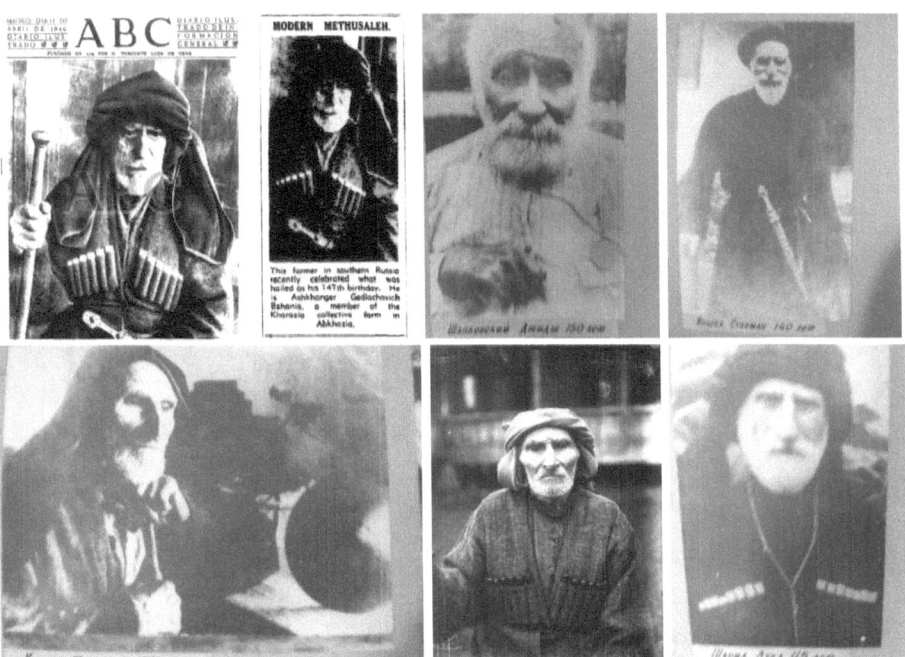

Diets and Lifestyles of the Worlds Oldest Peoples

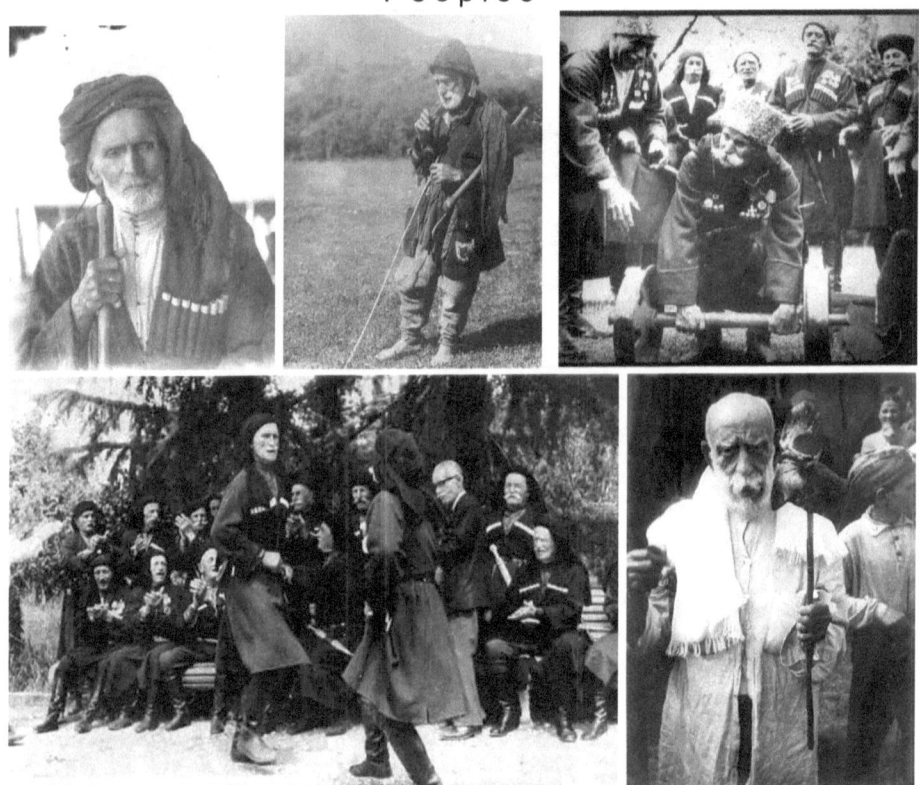

I had a long talk with this diminutive - she stands not five feet tall - sprightly woman who claimed to be 141 years old. . . . Although she carried a handsomely carved wooden walking stick, her nimbleness belied need of it. Her memory seemed excellent. . . . She spoke lucidly and easily about events recent and past. At the age of 75 to 80 as a midwife she assisted more than 100 babies into the world. . . . She described the life of women: "Women had a very difficult time before the Revolution; we were practically slaves." And she ended our talk with a toast, "I want to drink to women all over the world . . . for them not to work too hard and to be happy with their families."

Though he was greatly impressed by this elderly lady's charm and spirit, Leaf did not simply take her word for her age. To the contrary, he went to significant efforts to assess it objectively. Such a task is harder than it might sound, for there are no signs in the human body, like the annual rings of a tree, that tell us a person's age.

After laborious investigations, Leaf concluded that Mrs. Lasuria was close to 130 years old. He wasn't certain about that, saying only that he had arrived at a degree of confidence and this was his best estimate. But he was sure of one thing. She was one of the oldest persons he had ever met.

Everywhere he went in Abkhazia, Leaf met elders in remarkable health. The area seemed to warrant its reputation as the mecca of super longevity. Like others who have studied the elders of Abkhazia, Leaf had colorful stories to tell. He wrote of one elder, nearly 100, whose hearing was still good and whose vision was still superb.

"Have you ever been sick?" Leaf asked.

The elder thought for some time, then replied, "Yes, I recall once having a fever, a long time ago."

"Do you ever see a doctor?"

The old man was surprised by the question, and replied, "Why should I?"

Leaf examined him and found his blood pressure to be normal at 118/60 and his pulse to be regular at 70 beats per minute.

"What was the happiest period of your life?" Leaf asked.

"I feel joy all my life. But I was happiest when my daughter was born. And saddest when my son died at the age of one year from dysentery."

Among the others Leaf met were a delightful trio of gentlemen who, like many elderly Abkhazians, were still working despite their advanced age. They were Markhti Tarkhil, whom Leaf believed to be 104; Temur Tarba, who was apparently 100; and Tikhed Gunba, a mere youngster at 98. All were born locally. Temur said his father died at 110, his mother at 104, and an older brother just that year at 109. After a short exam, Leaf said that Temur's blood pressure was a youthful 120/84, and his pulse was regular at a rate of 69.

The old fellows clowned around constantly, joking and teasing each other and Leaf. While he was checking pulses and blood pressures the other two would shake their heads in mock sadness at the one being examined, saying "Bad, very bad!" They never seemed to tire of friendly joking, always finding new ways to have fun. Leaf was impressed by their sharp minds, high spirits, and relentless sense of humor.

Like many of the elders in Abkhazia, regardless of the weather, these men swam daily in cold mountain streams. One day, Leaf accompanied Markhti Tarkhil on his morning plunge and was astonished by the vitality and physical agility of the 104-year-old. It was a steep and rugged half-mile climb down from the road to the river, but Markhti moved with confident speed and agility. Seeing Markhti take off down the slope, Leaf, a physician coming from a society where elders have thin and fragile bones, was concerned that the older man might fall, and thought he should accompany Markhti down the hill and see to it that he didn't slip. But he was unable to do so, because he couldn't keep up with the pace of the far older man, who as it turned out never lost his footing. Later, Leaf learned from the regional doctor that there is no osteoporosis among the active elders, and that fractures are rare.

When Markhti arrived at the riverbank, he stripped and waded out into the stream, immersing his entire body in the cold water. A young guide Leaf had brought with him from Moscow also stripped and began wading into the water, but immediately jumped out, exclaiming that the water was far too cold.

After bathing in the cold water for some time, Markhti got out, dried himself off, put on his clothes, and proceeded to climb swiftly back up the rugged slope, with Leaf, who was a half-century younger and who considered himself physically fit, once again struggling to keep up.

Are They Really That Old?

After Leaf's articles in National Geographic appeared, however, a heated controversy developed over the validity of the ages claimed by some Abkhazians. When people say they are 140 or 150 years old, this naturally raises eyebrows. When the Soviet press announced that Shirali Muslimov was 168 years old, and the government commemorated the assertion by putting his face on a postage stamp, knowledgeable scientists around the world were skeptical.

How old, in fact, are the oldest Abkhazians? No one knows with absolute certainty. In the days when these elders were born, probably less than one-tenth of 1 percent of the world's population was keeping written birth records. When birth records are lacking or questionable, as they are in almost all cases of people born prior to 1920 in regions like the Caucasus, contemporary researchers have had to be creative in developing methods to appraise the ages of elders. Many volumes have been written about the enterprising techniques that have been employed in the effort, and probably an equal number of scholarly volumes have been written critiquing these techniques. It has been a difficult task.

Probably the foremost skeptic about the extremely old ages sometimes claimed for elders in the Caucasus was a geneticist from Soviet Georgia named Zhores A. Medvedev, an expert in the methodologies used in the effort to arrive at accurate age verifications in Abkhazia and elsewhere in the Caucasus. Medvedev's articles expressing his doubts received a great deal of attention when they were published in the scientific journal The Gerontologist shortly after Leaf's articles appeared in National Geographic. (Gerontology is the study of the changes and associated problems in the mind and body that accompany aging.) In these articles, Medvedev presented convincing evidence that the claims that people were regularly living past the age of 120 were not to be trusted. At the same time, though, he recognized that unusual longevity in the region was a genuine reality, and that the area was indeed home to an inordinate number of extremely healthy elders.

My interest in longevity in Abkhazia, however, doesn't depend on whether any specific individuals have reached ages beyond 120. Perhaps none have, but I don't find the question to be particularly important. What makes these people fascinating to me is the fact that an extraordinary percentage of Abkhazians have lived to ripe old ages while retaining their full health and vigor. What I find remarkable is the high degree of physical and mental fitness commonly found among the elders in Abkhazia, and their obvious joy in life.

****

What do these really old people in Abkhazia eat? Let's find out...

Diets and Lifestyles of the Worlds Oldest Peoples

Abkhazia Diet

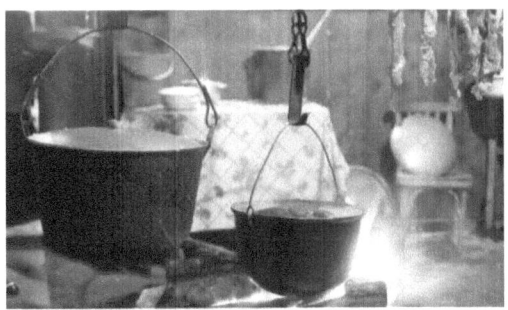

Much of the information on the Abkhazia Diet is taken from the article "Nutrition for Longevity by Dr. Farid Alakbarli (Alakbarli)

The typical diet of Azerbaijani villagers consists primarily of eggs, cheese, butter, yogurt, milk, curds (shor), sour cream, bread, various vegetables, fruits and herbs. They are used to eating soup made of yogurt and greens (dovgha) along with various soups made with beans, peas and grains. In the olden days, people who enjoyed longevity did not eat very much bread or products made of flour.

Animal Fat Consumption
Historically, Azerbaijanis eat fairly large amounts of animal fat,

which is considered by modern scientists to be the "No. 1 Killer."

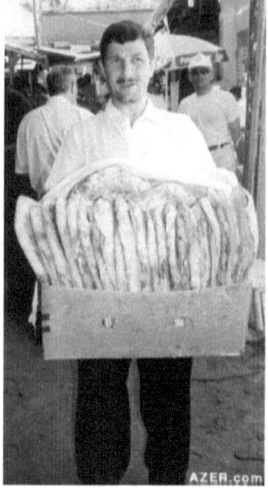

Why then has this slayer not visited upon the centenarians from

villages of the Lerik district in Azerbaijan, where quite a number of residents live beyond 120 years old?

Animal fat is fairly harmless to Azerbaijanis because they follow nutritional guidelines set forth by the physicians of medieval Azerbaijan who insisted that there is no such thing as completely healthy or unhealthy foodstuffs. Rather, these properties are determined a great deal by the quantity that is consumed and the way food is combined.

For example, according to the "Book of Medicine" (Tibbnama, 1712) you can consume animal fat, but you shouldn't overdo it, and you must counter the effects of fat by eating fresh vegetables and greens like spinach, celery, dill, onions, spring onions, coriander, mint, basil, tarragon and parsley. Modern scientists confirm that the food fibers contained in green vegetables and herbs decrease the assimilation of fats in the stomach.

Diets and Lifestyles of the Worlds Oldest Peoples

According to modern scientific medicine, animal fat, in fact, must be consumed (though in moderation), as it is necessary for creating hormones and promoting the normal functioning of the liver, heart and brain. If we examine the teeth of a human being, we notice that they contain features typical to both carnivorous and herbivorous beings.

Above: Traditional Tandir bread is wide and flat and made by hand. At Taza Bazaar in downtown Baku.

This fact proves that our early ancestors ate meat, and that the human organism is historically adapted to the consumption of animal fat. However, along with meat, early humans ate large amounts of vegetables and fruits. Medieval Azerbaijani physicians proposed the same approach: Don't eat just meat. Don't eat just vegetables. Eat both and combine them correctly! As opposed to one-sided theories of the modern day, such as vegetarianism, the medieval approach is based on their observation of the biological nature of the human being.

A high level of animal fat consumption is not just limited to longevity in Azerbaijan. Fifteen years ago, correspondents from the Russian magazine "Vokrug Sveta" (Around the World) interviewed elderly people in Abkhazia and questioned them about their diet. It turned out that most of the centenarians enjoyed fatty meat, preferably lamb. As distinct from Azerbaijanis, Georgians drank wine even at the age of 100. However, most people who enjoy longevity in the Caucasus don't eat very much meat in the first place, and they habitually consume large amounts of yogurt as well as vegetables and fruits to neutralize the negative effects of animal fat.

In addition to yogurt and garlic, it is also possible to counter the negative effect of fats with liberal amounts of raw onion, lemon juice, pomegranate juice and with the traditional burgundy- colored, sour spice known as sumag. These all work to promote digestion and break up the fat.

<u>Honey or Sugar?</u>

Even though Azerbaijani cuisine is rich in sweets, traditionally, Azerbaijanis didn't overuse them. When preparing national sweets like pakhlava, shakarbura and halva, they preferred honey over sugar. For example, the Azerbaijani scientist Yusif Khoyi in his "Baghdad's Collection" recommends preparing jams and sweets with honey. Modern science has established that honey contains vitamins, ferments and is considerably healthier than sugar. According to Professor M. Sultanov, the regular use of honey and the avoidance of sugar contribute to health and long life.

Professor John Yudkin of London University points out: "Not fat, but sugar leads to coronary heart disease-the sugar that you pour in coffee or tea, or eat with cakes, sweets or chocolate."

Sugar, if used excessively, turns to fat and cholesterol in the organism. Previously, poor people in the rural areas of Azerbaijan considered sugar as a delicacy and used it only on rare occasions. The standard fare for peasants included dairy products and herbs, not sweets. As for rich people, they preferred honey. According to recipes from the "Tibbnama", all kinds of Azerbaijani halva should be prepared on the basis of honey. Therefore, the harmful influence of "the white killer" that we struggle against in modern society was avoided.

Modern man might think: "Why buy expensive honey, when it's possible to substitute sugar that is much cheaper?" Unfortunately, most of the national desserts in modern Azerbaijan are based on sugar now. But in the long run, such economics are injurious to human health. Muhammad Husein-khan (18th century) also points out that the regular consumption of honey diluted with water prolongs human life. Nevertheless, even though honey is better than sugar, it should not be overused.

Yogurt and Longevity
Since antiquity it was believed that regular consumption of yogurt is the secret to longevity, as it promotes digestion and rejuvenates the organism. The "Tibbnama" recommends adding yogurt to cooked dishes. To promote digestion of meat, it was suggested to serve it with yogurt sprinkled with mint. If you eat yogurt on its own, add chopped garlic.

In Azerbaijan, a popular drink (ayran) is made by diluting salted yogurt with water. This drink is known to lower blood pressure and treat diarrhea. The word "yogurt" itself is of Turkic (Azerbaijani and Turkish) origin and derived from the verb "yogurmak" - "to knead." The medical effect of yogurt is explained by the fact that it contains useful micro-organisms such as lactobacteria.

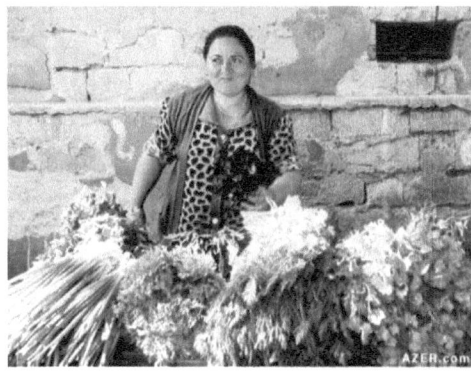

Above: At the bazaar, a woman sells greens such as green onion,

dill, cilantro and a purple variety of basil. Vegetables and fresh herbs play an important role in Azerbaijani cuisine.

Since the accumulation of waste substances in the in inflammation of the bowels is harmful to all organs of an organism, normal digestion of food contributes to a healthy and long life. Modern scientists in Japan have also established that regular consumption of yogurt protects the organism from the injurious influence of radioactive rays and prevents the development of cancer.

Garlic - Elixir of Youth

The healing properties of garlic are often mentioned in books by numerous ancient authors throughout the region-in Azerbaijan, Arabia, Persia, Tibet and China. According to the "Tibbnama", regular consumption of garlic prevents gray hair, strengthens memory and eyesight and is good for the heart. In Tibet, an herbal potion of garlic and spirits was known as an "elixir of youth." In Azerbaijan, physicians used infusions of garlic and saffron in their spirits.

Modern scientists confirm that the regular consumption of garlic lowers the level of cholesterol in the organism and improves the circulation of blood. As a result, all organs are well supplied with blood. For example, a proper supply of blood to the head prevents hair from graying, refreshes the face and improves memory. When blood is able to circulate well in the heart vessels, it prevents myocardial infarction.

Azerbaijanis have combined these two foods - garlic and yogurt - which are typical to diets of people who enjoy the benefits of long life. They chop garlic and add it to yogurt in a dish called "sarimsagli gatig" (yogurt with garlic). The "Tibbnama" also suggests mixing garlic with yogurt. This combination is used as a condiment with dishes made of flour or meat, such as dolma of grape leaves (stuffed grape leaves), khash, khingal and others.

Limit Bread

The excessive use of bread so typical to modern Azerbaijan cuisine can be traced to the influence of Russian cuisine. In the past Azerbaijanis did not overuse bread and flour products. They never had what might be called a cult of bread. Pilaf was never eaten along with bread because rice was considered to be a substitute for wheat. But these days, many people eat pilaf with bread, and also with national dishes made with dough, such as khingal, gurza, arishta, dushbara, umaj and others.

Physicians of medieval Azerbaijan didn't recommend eating much bread, especially on hot summer days. Modern investigations prove that overuse of bread, desserts and carbohydrates promotes the creation of cholesterol in the organism and leads to coronary disease and obesity. They concluded that overuse of bread is more dangerous than the regular consumption of animal fat.

Note that the national Azerbaijani bread (chorak) does not resemble Russian bread: it is a thin, flat bread, not a round loaf. Another national substitution for bread is lavash, a paper-thin bread - neither of these two types is very heavy to digest when eaten in moderation.

Use of Herbs

Since antiquity, Azerbaijanis have been convinced that saffron and licorice prolong life, refresh the skin and face, and promote health for the liver, heart and kidneys. In addition, persons of longevity traditionally consume large amounts of vegetables and fruits, including apples.

The Azerbaijani physician Yusif Ibn Ismayil Khoyi (1311) wrote: "If eaten regularly, apples rejuvenate the organism, strengthening the heart, stomach, liver, intestine and stimulating the appetite. Regular use of apples prevents heavy breathing and excessive heartbeat in elderly persons. Apples refresh the brain and strengthen its efficiency."

Fruits, vegetables, various wild medicinal plants and products prepared from them - jams, juices, sharbats, wines, dried fruits and spices - all play an important role in Azerbaijan's national cuisine. In particular, hot dishes are combined with various vegetables, fruits, greens and spices.

Modern investigations show that vegetables and fruits contain many micro-elements, vitamins and fibers that neutralize cholesterol. Of course, scientists in the Middle Ages had no knowledge about these substances, but based on close observation, they drew similar conclusions that are being confirmed by modern scientific research.

Tea, Not Coffee

Regular consumption of tea is another main characteristic of people who enjoy long life in Azerbaijan. According to Muhammad Husein-khan (18th century), tea is a healthier beverage than coffee. He points out that: "Tea is a diuretic. It alleviates headaches caused by spasms and cold. In addition, tea cleanses the blood, stomach and brain and refreshes the face. If used moderately, it can treat rapid heartbeat, facilitate regular breathing and is good for the heart. This drink eases melancholy, sorrow and bad spirits."

Modern investigations prove that tea promotes longevity. It contains caffeine, which stimulates the nervous system, and theophylline, which enlarges blood vessels, eliminates spasms and improves the function of the heart. It also contains tannins, which strengthen blood vessels and prevent bleeding. As distinct from coffee, tea not only does not increase the risk of the myocardial infarction but even lowers it, because theophylline enlarges the blood vessels of the heart.

However, one should avoid drinking tea on an empty stomach and should not drink it very hot. Milk neutralizes the negative effects of caffeine. Even though tea mixed with milk is considered to be healthier, it is not popular in Azerbaijan. Tea is historically cultivated in the Lankaran district of Azerbaijan, which curiously enough, is a region known for its longevity.

<u>Cheap, Healthy Food</u>
Although the famous Azerbaijani Oil Baron Haji Zeynalabdin Taghiyev (1823-1924) enjoyed a very long life span, most elderly people in Azerbaijan are not so well off. When analyzing their diet, we see that they eat relatively cheap foods: eggs, yogurt, vegetables, fruits and beans. In addition, most of them don't overeat. Nor are they overweight because they are involved with hard physical labor.

In the past, those who enjoyed long life in our country rarely consumed the expensive dishes of our national cuisine, except on special occasions. Baked goods, kababs, pilaf seasoned with meat and dried fruits were usually reserved for the New Year celebration (Novruz), Muslim religious festivals (such as Gurban Bayram) and wedding celebrations. During the 19th century, even wealthy landowners didn't eat sweets and meat every day because it was considered to be harmful.

Most people in Azerbaijan who enjoy the benefits of longevity actually know nothing about cholesterol, carbohydrates or vegetarianism. They simply maintain the nutritional practices of their fathers and grandfathers, who lived to be more than 100 years old. This reality would seem to prove that Azerbaijan's traditional diet, which has been tried and tested over centuries and millennia, is at least equal to modern theories of healthy nutrition, and may even be superior.

****

Next we move to Ecuador where a special "Vallay of Longevity" exists

Diets and Lifestyles of the Worlds Oldest Peoples

Vilcabamba Lifestyle

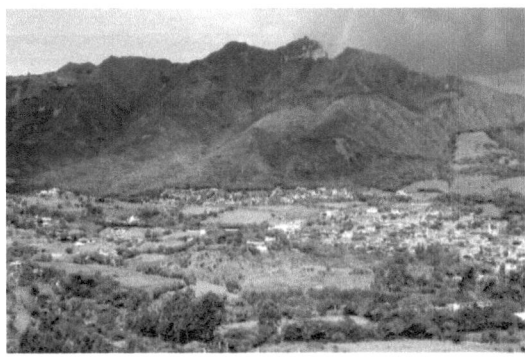

In 1970, scientists researching the link between diet and heart disease visited the small town of Vilcabamba, located high in the Ecuadorian Andes. The scientists included Dr. Alexander Leaf of Harvard Medical School, Dr. Harold Elrick of the University of California at San Diego, and a group from the University of Quito.

The scientists found that the residents of Vilcabamba, who were principally of European descent, had very low cholesterol levels and very few of them ever suffered from heart disease. But more remarkable was the longevity of the Vilcabambans. Many of the town residents claimed to be over 100 years old. A few of them stated their age as being over 140 years old. These ages appeared to be confirmed by birth and baptismal records.

As word of Vilcabamba's "longevos" (very old people) got out, the town became an international sensation. Numerous articles promoted the town as a Shangri-la whose residents -- blessed with extraordinary health and longevity -- lived in closer harmony with nature, untouched by the stresses of modern life. Appropriately, Vilcabamba meant "Sacred Valley" in the Inca language.

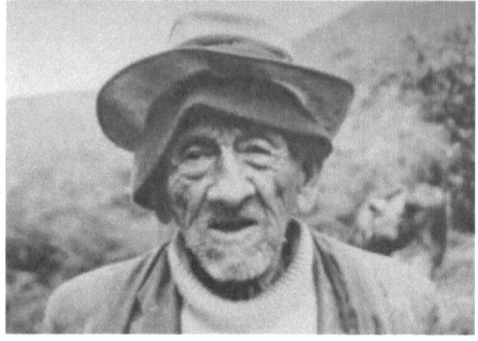

Gabriel Erazo claimed to be 132 years old. He also always wore two hats.

Halsell's picturesque account of life in Vilcabamba emphasized the simple virtues of the villager's way of life. She wrote, "I lived in a dirt-floor mountain hut with Gabriel Erazo, who matter-of-factly says, 'I am 132.'" Halsell described how Erazo stayed healthy by composing poetry in his head while hiking in the mountains. She also wrote of 113-year-old Gabriel Sanchez who "climbed the steep El Chaupi mountain to work all day with his crude hoe or lampa, cultivating a small plot of ground."

Several books published in the mid-1970s further enhanced the town's reputation. In 1975, Dr. David Davies, an English gerontologist, published (Davies, 1975) about his research in Vilcabamba.

There is also the "magical" water they drink:

High up among the surrounding mountain peaks lies an area of primeval tundra, which is made up of great masses of vegetation .... layer upon layer of these grasses and vegetation of many types and colors. In this untouched and uninhabited area, there are also some fourteen lakes, each containing the melt of this uncontaminated glacier ice.

This icy melt is often referred to as "Glacial Milk", a solution of ionically dissolved elements in a suspension of finely ground rock dust from the living parent rock of the mountains through glacial friction. The suspended minerals in this "Glacial Milk" are referred to as metallic colloidal minerals.

Come the rainy season, these lakes of glacial water overflow and flood the tundra, which then acts as a filter for any undesirable heavy metals or minerals. But this humic layer does far more than merely act as a filtering devise. These plants and ancient vegetation had never been exposed to any chemicals, fertilizers or pesticides. The plants are gradually transformed into humus, a rich organic mass that is food for new plant life.

After seeping through these countless layers of humic tundra, this purest of waters flows down into thousands of pools, then into hundreds of cascading waterfalls. And remember this part for a little later, because the countless waterfalls contribute to the extremely high negative ion count in the valley. Finally, the long journey of the pristine Agua Sacrada ends up in the water jugs and homes of the people of Vilcabamba.

They lead active, hard-working lifestyles.

The people of Vilcabamba don't exercise. They don't have to. Almost all of the area's residents are farmers. And the often rugged terrain requires them to hike up the slopes to pick fruits and till the soil on sloping hillsides.

They lead simple lives and have very little stress. The elderly are treated with great respect, and it's considered an honor to have reached old age.

When you lay it all out there, it's a simple formula really. Keep things natural and simple. Put good in, get good out. Work hard. Play hard. And respect your elders. These are the things that have drawn decades of expats to Vilcabamba. But unfortunately many have brought their old habits with them.

Stores now stock many packaged and processed foods. Drug and alcohol abuse are at an all time high among natives, and obesity has found its way onto the town's short list of medical concerns. The locals welcome foreigners and even some of their advancements, but many hope more of them will start to help keep this little-known paradise closer to the way they found it.

In order to properly digest the released nutrients, even with proper chewing, the hydrochloric acid content in the stomach has to be awfully strong. That means maintaining a pH somewhere between 1 and 3. And that, my friends, means having a VERY high acidic level. So how do healthy elders pull this off, while keeping their bodies balanced with a sufficient alkaline content? It's the water!

Laboratory analysis of the Vilcabamba water determined that the unique balance of enriched colloidal minerals in the local drinking water was ideal for promoting optimum human health. (1)

Note the high pH factor:

- ph factor 7.2
- total solids 262 mg
- hydrogen-bicarbonate (HCO2) 136.4
- hardness 140
- calcium 40.8
- magnesium 79.3
- chlorides 10.8
- sulphates 39
- potassium 1.2

- iron 0.03

Now, take a look at the list of the mineral content on the label of the bottled water you are drinking. Does it measure up to what is found in the Vicabamba water? If not, then you are being improperly nourished by the water you are drinking …. If not being outright poisoned!   At least for now and some time to come, Vilcabamba has a good source of clean, sweet water to nourish its inhabitants. This is, unfortunately, not the case in many parts of the world.

****

If you find yourself in Vilcabamba--What should you eat? That's up next…

Diets and Lifestyles of the Worlds Oldest Peoples

Vilcabamba Diet

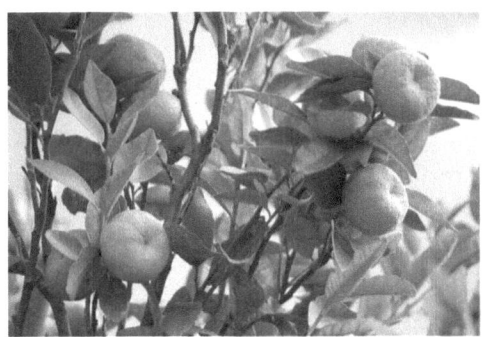

We mentioned the rivers that flow into Vilcabamba, providing water even for the dry season. The year-round availability of pure water allows the town's growing season to span pretty much the entire year. When leaving the tundra, the water also carries with it humus, an organic matter than serves as nutrients for the plants that are grown in the village. As a result, the area's produce has some of the highest antioxidant content in the world.

Keep in mind that Vilcabamba was almost completely unknown to the world until a few decades ago. In fact, until the 1960's, there wasn't even a road that led into the valley. As a result, the area has been protected from "civilization" and a lot of its vices. Chemical additives have never been a part of the area's farming. And, until recently, no packaged or prepared foods could be found on its grocery store shelves.

Residents of Vilcabamba have traditionally enjoyed a diet of fresh produce, whole grains, seeds, and nuts. They eat little fat and almost no animal products.

The book "An Operations Manual for Human Kind" By Paul Patrick Robinson (Robinson, 2011) contains a lot of information about the Vilcabamba diet:

When they prepare a salad they often toss in a few slices of mandarin oranges that grow in such abundance in this valley. The mandarin oranges not only enhance the flavor of the lettuce, but the vitamin C content helps their bodies absorb the iron in the leafy green vegetables. You will also see them mixing some local tomatoes with their broccoli. They have done so down through the ages, this food combining secret passed along from mother to daughter. Now, modern science has proven that these two foods taken together are potent cancer-fighters. Another "secret" ingredient in the Vilcabamban diet is avocado … think guacamole. Once again scientists have shown, after the fact, that the Old People of Vilcabamba were practicing some excellent natural medicine in their plentiful use of avocado in their diet. The natural oil of the avocado works synergistically with the leafy vegetables to maximize the nutrient value of the salad. The medicinal value of culturally traditional foods has always been a part of "folk wisdom" in places where the Centenarians thrive.

Quinoa is called the Queen of Grains. This is cheating a bit. Quinoa, like a number of other exotic grains, isn't really a grain at all … it is technically a fruit. In Botanical terms, quinoa is a pseudo-cereal along with amaranth and teff. It has grown in The Andes Mountains for more than 4,000 years. The Incas called quinoa "the Mother Grain" as eating this food tended to be nurturing and guarantee long life. It is used as a substitute for other grains like rice because of it's cooking characteristics.

The quinoa grown in Vilcabamba and surrounding Ecuadorian valleys is a variety called Altiplano, which simply can't be grown in the lower elevations of North America. The quinoa that you are probably used to finding in your local health food store is a brownish, bitterer tasting variety called "Sea Level quinoa." You can find the high altitude quinoa if you look for it, and it's worth the search.

In keeping with the Vilcabambanos use of raw or lightly cooked foods, uncooked seeds are added to soups and stews just as you would with barley or rice. Quinoa seeds absorb water very quickly and become as soft and chewy as cooked rice when added to soups. The seeds also cook very quickly at low temperatures, in only 15 minutes. This is one reason that Ecuadorians call quinoa "little rice."

Quinoa is one of the few foods that has an almost perfect balance of all eight essential amino acids, thus its use as a protein. It was used by the Incan armies in a mixture of quinoa and fat that they called "war balls" to sustain their energy during forced marches at high altitude. So if you want an energy boost and a super-healthy whole grain replacement, enjoy gluten-free South American Quinoa.

Perhaps this is one reason that the centenarians of Vilcabamba have almost always had a diet that was 70-75% uncooked, with an emphasis on salads, vegetables and locally grown fruits. Thus, they remain lean and hardy, not obese and sick.

The Vilcabambanos do cook their lentil beans, and probably so should you unless they are sprouted for salads. One of the types of beans most consumed is the black bean, sometimes called Spanish or Venezuelan beans. This variety of bean is exceptionally nutritious, containing within its dark coating phytonutrients and flavonoids that work together with the natural vitamins to help reduce some of the oxygen-related damage that can occur at higher altitudes. Black beans also contain about 185 milligrams of omega-3 fatty acids per cup, which is about three times most other varieties. It is a nutrient-dense food that goes perfectly with the low caloric intake of the local people.

Their use of natural, organic, unpasteurized yogurt from both goats and cows also provides the beneficial probiotics that might be heated out of the food. It goes without saying that keeping beneficial bacteria levels high in the intestinal tract is one of the best defenses against any pathogens that might be associated with eating "raw" foods.

****

From my research, the Hunza people of Northern Pakistan maybe the healthiest and longest lived community in the world. Let's learn about them next..

Diets and Lifestyles of the Worlds Oldest Peoples

Hunza Lifestyle

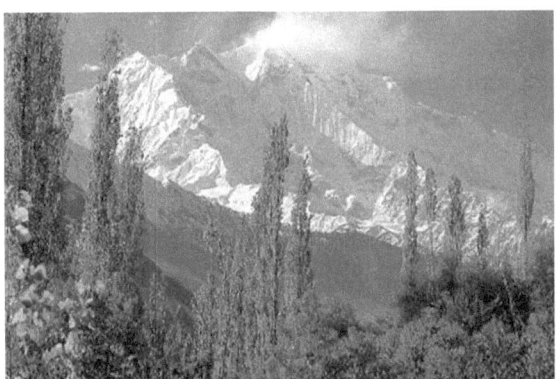

The 5 Secrets of The Hunza People to Live to 100
These good life choices will make you live longer, just ask the Hunza Tribe

All this time we thought that living forever would be down to cryogenics when in fact, it's taking it back to ancient ways. It's possible to live long and prosper right now.

How long do the Hunza people live?

You may have heard a lot of 'Hunza hype' recently because scientists are fascinated with the Hunza Tribe and with good reason. The Hunza live in the northern mountainous region of Pakistan and not only do they often surpass their hundredth birthday but their average life expectancy is around 120 years.

More importantly, they're all smiling and brimming with vitality. Their population is exceptionally fit and predominantly disease-free, irrespective of age. The Hunza valley women are renowned for their beauty and some can even fertile until after the age of 60, whilst the global population's long-term health is on the decline, hence why the western world is so keen to learn their secret.

Diets and Lifestyles of the Worlds Oldest Peoples

Secret No 1. An anti-inflammatory diet

Hunza people eat a highly effective anti-inflammatory diet of naturally grown ancient grains, raw fruits and vegetables, and lesser quantities of meat. Their strong immunity and low disease rate has been repeatedly linked to their high consumption of vitamin B-17, found in apricot kernels. We can certainly mimic their anti-inflammatory diet, we can even set up a subscription to the world's purest glacier water. But before we all go on a Whole Foods snatch n' grab mission, it's worth considering what else makes the Hunza people live longer and healthier lives.

Secret No 2. Social health

Congrats on the excellent 10k time and you're deadlifting like a dream but how's your 360 health? How the Hunza people live happy and healthy long lives can be largely attributed to their superior emotional state, living in peace and within a close-knit community. The McKinsey Report aptly refers to this broader definition of health as "adding life to our years", because there's no win in adding on the years if they're not spent in happiness. Social health refers to meaningful connection, forming nurturing relationships and reciprocal support. Research shows that loneliness and isolation can be just as damaging to a person's health as smoking 15 cigarettes a day.

Secret No 3. Spiritual Health

Scientists have identified other dimensions of health every bit as important as the physical. Spiritual health is integrating meaning and purpose into your life makes you feel rooted, mindful and present. US scientists have distinguished a link between greater purpose and a lesser probability of suffering a stroke.

Secret No 4. Calmness saves lives

Mental health goes far deeper than just your happiness barometer, it's your ability to adapt, memory recall, process emotions and apply logic to situations. Chronic stress and anxiety has been proven by Yale University to shorten your lifespan so mitigate that to retain the years.

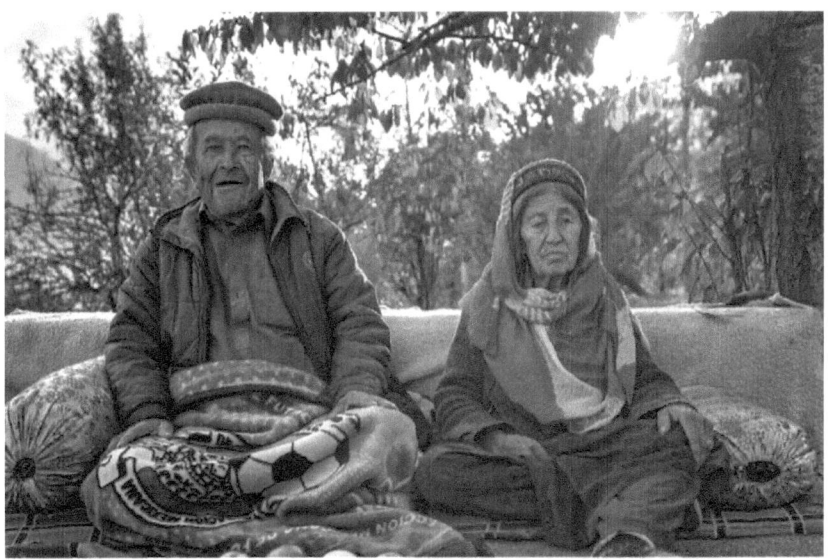

Secret No 5. Amp up your immunity

Research from the World Economic Forum shows that globally, we're living longer than ever before but spending more of those years in poor health. Chronic disease is on the rise; conditions like arthritis, dementia, diabetes and obesity that won't necessarily kill us, but will compromise our quality of life.

And yes--Of course we want to know what the Hunzas eat...

Diets and Lifestyles of the Worlds Oldest Peoples

Hunza Diet

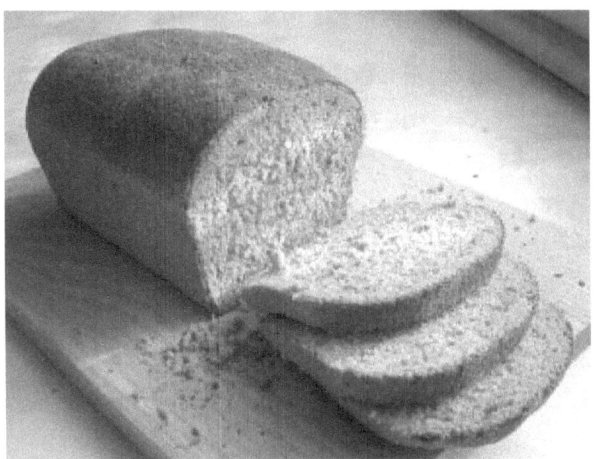

What the Hunzakuts thrive on, mostly, is the famous Hunza Bread. This is made from a coarse, whole grain, barley flour and water and formed into a kind of pancake. Remember, this is WHOLE GRAIN, hand-ground and fresh from a clean highly fertile land.   In addition, they also eat a lot of vegetables, green leaves, fruits, grain and some nuts. Their grain selection includes wheat, barley, buckwheat, corn, millet, alfalfa, and rye. Their vegetables are mostly potatoes, tomatoes, carrots, onions, garlic, peas, beans and pulses. The fruits that are generally available in the region are mulberries, apricots, apples, cucumbers, grapes, peaches, cherries and some melons. It's an excellent variety that appears to supply all essential vitamins in precise quantities.

The diet of these people was studied by Pakistani nutritionist, Dr. S. Maqsood. He found the average caloric intake of the Hunzakuts to be about 1900 (about 2/3 that of an average American). 98 1/2% of this consisted of protein, fat and carbohydrates "from vegetable sources." The food originating in animal flesh or from dairy products comprised only about 1 1/2% of their total food intake. And, this amount is calculated from an average consumption. That means that the animal by-products part of the diet is not consistent, but rather sporadic causing little continual damage.

The most important single observation to be made about food consumption in Hunzaland is that almost everything is eaten raw, uncooked, and just as nature intended. This preference for live food includes every kind of sprout (one of the most 'living' sources of nutrition known).

In summary then, the people of Hunza eat almost nothing in the way of meat, dairy products, eggs, animal fats or processed and chemicalized foods. The only exceptions to this come with what is now being brought into the area from the outside, as "progress" makes its unhealthy advance on the people of this peaceful mountain region.

What we have outlined here appears to be the latest craze in 'healthy diets' in the U.S., but, in fact is the classic "Hunza Health Recipe." Our third Health Commandment then is based upon the knowledge that a community (which exists today) is surviving in a much more healthy way because they have followed (more closely) the diet that the Creator intended for us. The Commandment is this, "Work in harmony with your earth so that it will yield foods for you that consist mainly of live, organically grown grains, seeds, vegetables and nuts. Eat these raw and don't tamper with the way they are given to you."

****

Now let's do comparison matrixes for all of these communities to compare lifestyles and diets side by side....

Lifestyle & Diet Recommendations

Before making specific diet suggestions based on these four long lived communities I decided to make a matrix of both cultural and dietary factors. These factors are rated (High-Medium-Low) Types of foods are also provided in the Diet Table.

Lifestyle Factors

Description	Okinawa	Abkhazia	Vilcabamba	Hunzas
Exercise	High	High	Medium	Very High
Naturally Pure Water	Medium	High	High	High
Sense of Community	High	High	High	High
Happiness	High	High	High	High
Spiritual Practices & Inner Peace	High	High	High	High
Respect for Elderly	High	High	High	High

Dietary Factors/Foods

Description	Okinawa	Abkhazia	Vilcabamba	Hunzas
Vegetables	High-Sweet Potatos, Goya (bitter melon), Shima Rakkyo, Okra, Handama, Carrots , radish, marrow, onions, carrots, cabbage and leafy greens, Soya, squash	High- string beans, corn, cabbage, tomatoes, spinach, celery, dill, onions, spring onions, coriander, mint, basil, tarragon and parsley	High-Potatos, Mayoko, Payoko	High-Tomatoes, onions, garlic, spinach, turnips, carrots, pumpkins, cabbage, and cauliflower
Legumes	High	High	High	High-beans, lentils
Meat/Fat	Low-Pork	Low-Lamb	Low	Minimal
Grains	Rice	Buckwheat	High-Trigo (Wheat), Rice	wheat, barley, buckwheat, corn, millet, alfalfa, and rye
Fish	Low	Low	Low	Minimal
Fruits	High-Watermellon, Pineapple, Mango, Papaya, Passion Fruit, Shiikwa	High-Apples, cherry plums, barberries, blackberries, pomegranates, green grapes, tomatoes	High-oranges, blackberries, papayas, bananas, figs, avocados, Citroen, Granadias	High-mulberries, apricots, apples, cucumbers, grapes, peaches, cherries and some melons
Nuts	Pine nuts	Achapa, Walnuts	High-macadamia nuts, almonds	Almonds, Beachnuts, Walnuts, Flax
Special Bread		High-Limit Bread		High-Hunza Bread
Sugars	Sugarcane (Unrefined)	Honey, Sugarbeets	Panela-(Unrefined Sugarcane)	Honey

Diets and Lifestyles of the Worlds Oldest Peoples

Other Common Foods		*Yogurt, Garlic*	*Quinoa*	*Yogurt*
Common Herbs		*Saffron, Licorice*		
Common Drinks	*High-Tumeric Tea*	*High-Tea, Mountain Waters*	*High-Mountain Waters (Glacial Milk)*	*High-Mountain Waters*
Number of Daily Meals				*Two*

From the above tables comparing lifestyles and diets here are my recommendations for the Longevity Diet which is taken from these real world examples:

1) Drink Pure Water--but not just bottled water but water with appropriate nutrients like the mountain streams provide to the long lived communities.

2) None of these communities are pure vegetarians but they all have very low levels of meat and fish--just because their traditional diets are oriented that way. Meat and Fish comprises only 1-3% of their daily diets

3) Two communities-- the Abkhazians and Hunzas eat natural grain, low fat, and high protein breads with fruit and nuts added. These are Limit Breads for the Abkhazians, and Hunza Breads for the Hunzas.

4) Several of the communities have lots of home grown fruits--of a variety of types. Eat lots of fruit.

5) Sugars are all natural or unrefined sugars whether from honey or from various types of fruits, or sugarcane.

6) They all consume high levels of legumes and vegetables. These types of food are the large majorities of their diets. (Greater than 65%)

7) The number of meals daily are only stated for the Hunzas who regularly eat two large meals daily. My research didn't tell me the number of meals in the other communities.

The Effect of Lifestyle Factors:

In the lifestyle factors table you can see a lot of parallels to the 10 Principles of Personal Longevity.

The principle longevity lifestyle factors I found from my research include:

- Lots of daily exercise--This ties into my previous research that exercise is one of the most critical factors in long term health.
- Naturally Pure Water with mountain nutrients-This was a surprise to me since I've heard others tout the benefits of water but never really gave it much serious consideration
- A strong Sense of Community- The community and happiness factors both illustrate the need for purpose and happiness to make our lives more fulfilling
- Overall Happiness
- Spiritual Practices & Inner Peace--A critical factor I've been teaching for years having earlier found that almost all super centenarians have these attributes which I believe help bring a spiritual blueprint of health down into our bodies
- Respect for Elderly--This relates a lot to the Principle of Life Purpose. People need meaning in their lives to go on living and being respected and asked for advice as an elderly person is important in making their lives worthwhile.

If you have read any of my other books on Longevity you will realize that these lifestyle factors are all part of what we already teach. They show some real world examples which further validate our 10 Principles approach.

****

Next lets look at a new Diet and Lifestyle Plan to apply what we have learned to ourselves…

Diets and Lifestyles of the Worlds Oldest Peoples

Diets and Lifestyles of the Worlds Oldest Peoples

A Longevity Diet & Lifestyle Plan

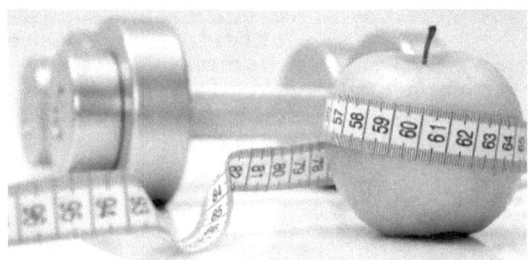

Changing your lifestyle and diet to a new permanent and healthier "standard" or "baseline" is not easy to do.

It is up to your motivation and willingness to follow these steps -- and get help from others to hold you accountable.

STEP #1:

Determine what your breakeven level of calories is per day. In other words how many calories can you eat daily without gaining any weight? Also determine how many calories you should eat daily in "weight loss mode".

An example table is below on general calorie levels need by sex and age:

Age and gender	Estimated calories for those who are not physically active	
	Total daily calorie needs*	Daily limit for empty calories
Children 2-3 yrs	1000 cals	135**
Children 4-8 yrs	1200-1400 cals	120
Girls 9-13 yrs	1600 cals	120
Boys 9-13 yrs	1800 cals	160
Girls 14-18 yrs	1800 cals	160
Boys 14-18 yrs	2200 cals	265
Females 19-30 yrs	2000 cals	260
Males 19-30 yrs	2400 cals	330
Females 31-50 yrs	1800 cals	160
Males 31-50 yrs	2200 cals	265
Females 51+ yrs	1600 cals	120
Males 51+ yrs	2000 cals	260

However, the above table may not apply to everyone based on your body type and metabolism.

I encourage you to work with a medical professional to carefully determine your daily caloric needs.

Once you have a good caloric number we can proceed to Step 2:

STEP #2:

Start changing what you drink to conform to longevity community guidelines.

For example--drink healthy pure water--like these old people do from their mountain streams. You may not have access to the streams but you do have access to lots of brands of pure water and you can get recommendations on additional mineral waters.

The Mayo Clinic has determined these average guidelines for the amount of water you should drink each day:

*The Institute of Medicine determined that an adequate intake
(AI) for men is roughly about 13 cups (3 liters) of total
beverages a day. The AI for women is about 9 cups (2.2
liters) of total beverages a day.*

<u>Stop drinking all sodas and other diet or sugary drinks. They are all
bad for you</u>

Most of us lived dehydrated and we should drink much more water
each day than we currently do.

<u>STEP #3:</u>

Start planning meals from the "Dietary Factors/Foods" Table which
lists many grains, nuts, and fruits which the long lived communities
each. This is in the Chapter titled " Lifestyle & Diet
Recommendations"

You should make these types of food the staples of your daily diet.

This includes the various breads like Hunza Bread--whose recipe is
given in the recipe chapter below.

The calorie intake you should plan for daily should be less than
your breakeven calorie intake. Your daily intake should be the
number your worked out with your health professional.

My doctor friend worked out the numbers for me to lose weight.
Since I'm a big guy she calculated that my breakeven value was
3600 calories per day. She recommended that I only consume
about 2800 calories per day while I was still trying to lose weight.

These numbers will be different for everyone--which is why you
should consult a medical and/or diet and nutrition professional.

I also decided to follow the Hunza practice of only eating two meals per day with snacks in between--this is just me--I'm not recommending that everyone eat two meails per day.

Another factor to consider are meats, poultry, and fish. You don't need to become a vegetarian but it is important to realize that most long lived communities only consume about 1-3% of their diet as meat, poultry, and fish.

Most of this long term healthy diet is going to be grains, nuts, and fruits--so you just need to get used to it.

STEP #4:

Daily Exercise is required. You must exercise everyday the rest of your life.

Let me elaborate--In all of my studies of long lived people well over 100 only two factors stood out:

* Daily exercise even into extreme old age

* Inner Peach and/or Spiritual Practices

Each of the communities we cover in this book also have lifestyles which involve heavy daily exercise--and no you don't get to quit when you reach 100 years old.

A basic rule of thumb I've learned is "If you want to live--keep exercising. If you want to die-Stop".

It doesn't have to be a huge amount of exercise daily. Maybe just a walk for 20 minutes.--but it has to be something.

You can work with a Personal Trainer to develop your own daily program if you don't know what to do yourself.

SO EXERCISE AND KEEP DOING IT FOREVER !

Step #5:

Once you have started to reduce your weight and lead a healthier lifestyle then you are ready for the next and biggest step---

Learn the 10 Principles of Personal Longevity and start applying them to your life.

These principles include many non physical factors which affect your overall health and teach you how to optimize your long term health.

Our training program is online and includes many videos, reading assignments, and exercises.

If you truly want to change your lifestyle, improve your longevity, and live with optimum long term health, then this training is for you.

****

In the next chapter we do a short review of the 10 Principles and provide information on where you can learn more....

What is Personal Longevity?

The Personal Longevity Program is the term I use to describe the implementation process of the 10 Principles of Personal Longevity which are listed below:

The 10 Principles of Personal Longevity

1) Real Long Lived Persons Exist
People really have lived a long time-so you can do it too
2) Define Your Purpose in Life
Know your life purpose-To live life with meaning
3) Enable Your Life Urge
Know without doubt that you will live a long and happy life
4) The Importance of a Spiritual Connection
A spiritual connection is important for happiness & long term health
5) Having Love in your Heart
Unconditional Love is is real-It will make you happier and healthier
6) Activate your Vital Forces
Improve the vitality of your energy body for health and to enjoy life more
7) The Science of Longevity
Use new therapies and discoveries from Science & Medicine
8) Keep your Physical Body Healthy
Eat a proper diet, use herbal supplements, and exercise
9) Use Your Intuition for Safety
Learn to use your intuition to keep you safe
10) Implement the above principles in your life
Implement these principles for long term health, greater happiness, and extended longevity

I developed these principles after a lifetime of experiences, learning, belonging to different spiritual and health organizations, and getting to know many persons in the longevity movement over the last five years.

The 10 Principles are a step by step philosophy of total health which covers our spirit, mind, vital forces, and physical body.

It is a comprehensive approach to how we can tune our lifestyle and ourselves to live in optimum total health which then also results in long term happiness and greater length of life.

By teaching people how to live by these principles we can bring together all of the best of holistic/alternative healing, and traditional medical practices in ways that nobody else is doing.

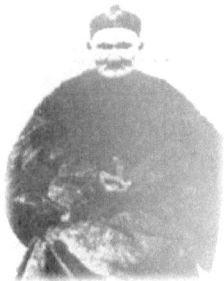

Principle #1 – The Reality of Long Lived People

The first principle is the evidence of people who have lived well over the age of 120 years old to 150-180-200, and even a 256 year old man from China: LI CHING-YUN: The Longest Lived person of record-256 Years (Source-The New York Times-May 6, 1933)

This principle is designed to help people break out of the bounds of their beliefs about how long we can all really live.

The Second Principle is all about Life Purpose

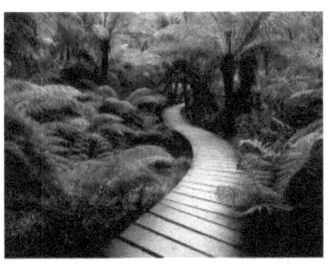

Within our Longevity Research we found out, that if one doesn't have a reason to live, or have a purpose in life–then what is the point?

This means a very important step to developing longevity is how you can develop your own positive life purpose, or bring it up to date with your phase in life. Without reviewing your purpose–none of the rest of the longevity principles matter.

I'm not going to get into all of the principles in detail here--since that is part of the Longevity Coaching training, but I wanted to give you the reader just a little flavor of what this subject is all about.

The Scope of this book is too limited to go into all of the 10 Principles in detail.

The best way to learn the principles is to take our Longevity Coaching training program which is entirely online.

Checkout the website at: http://personal-longevity.com for more details and signup for the email list on the right side of the page to get four FREE videos on the Secrets of Longevity and Longevity Coaching

****

Finally, we present some traditional recipes from these long lived communities which you may want to make part of your regular new diet…

Diets and Lifestyles of the Worlds Oldest Peoples

Longevity Diet Recipes

Here is a collection of food preparation tips and recipes we found as part of our research on longevity communities:

A) Okinawan Recipes:

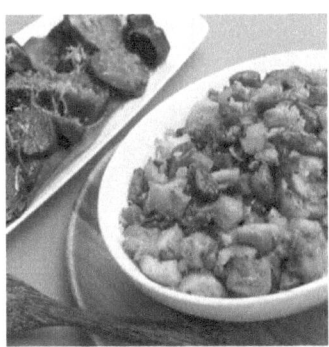

Okinawa Sweet Potatos

Ingredients

4 pounds Okinawa (purple) sweet potatoes or white sweet potatoes, scrubbed

2 limes

1/4 cup butter

Hawaiian red clay salt or sea salt

Preparation

1. Bring a large pot of water to a boil over high heat. Prick sweet potatoes with a fork and boil until tender when pierced, 30 to 35 minutes. Drain.

2. While potatoes are boiling, grate zest from limes and set aside; then squeeze juice from limes and set aside.

3. When potatoes are cool enough to handle, peel and slice into 1/2-in.-thick slices. Arrange on a platter, cover with foil, and put in a 200° oven to keep warm.

4. Melt butter in a small saucepan over medium heat until foaming. Stir in zest and cook until fragrant, 1 minute. Remove from heat and stir in lime juice. Drizzle lime butter over potatoes and sprinkle with salt.

Note: Nutritional analysis is per serving.

Note:

Okinawa sweet potatoes, also called purple sweet potatoes, are available at some Asian-food markets, farmers' markets, or online.

Goya Champuru--A cultural heritage of Okinawa

Ingredients

- 80 to 100 grams Pork
- 1 Bitter melon
- 300 grams Tofu (firm)
- 1 large Beaten egg
- 1 dash Dashi stock granules

- 1 tsp   * Miso
- 2 tsp   * Cooking sake
- 2 tbsp Soy sauce
- 1Bonito flakes

Method

1 Cut the bitter gourd in half lengthwise, and scrape out the white fluffy pith with a spoon. Slice into half-moon slices about 5 mm thick. Bring water to a boil in a pan, and briskly parboil the sliced bitter melon.

2 Drain the boiled bitter melon well. Heat oil in the pan and stir-fry the pork. When it's about halfway cooked, add the bitter melon and stir-fry.

3 When the bitter melon has wilted, add the tofu, miso, and cooking sake. Mix and stir-fry while lightly breaking up the tofu.

4 Pour in the beaten egg. When it's soft-set, mix it in. Add the dashi stock granules and drizzle in the soy sauce. Sprinkle on bonito flakes and it's done.

5 In Okinawa, they have a type of tofu called shima-dofu (island tofu) which is perfect for stir fries. It's hard to obtain outside Okinawa, so use firm tofu.

6 I used coarsely chopped pork offcuts this time, but I also recommend using pork belly slices.

7 I don't like the unique bitterness of bitter melon too much so I parboil it in Step 1, but if you like the bitterness, you can omit that step!

B) Abkhazia Recipes:

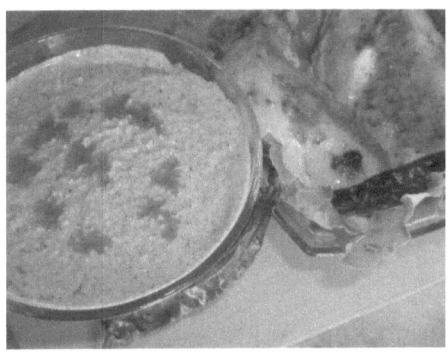

Arashykh Syzbal is an Abkhazian sauce similar to *bazhe sauce* but made with *ajika*. It is eaten with fried or boiled chicken or turkey. It is also used as a sauce for Abkhazian 'abysta', which is similar to *'gomi'* (Georgian: ღომი).

Ingredients: 300 grams of walnuts, 4 cloves of garlic, 1 tbs of *Ajika* (click link for recipe), 1 tbs of *Akhkhyla*(Abkhazian spice mix – click link for recipe), and salt.

Preparation: Grind the walnuts and garlic together.

Re-grind the ground walnuts and garlic.

Add 1 tbs of Ajika, 1 tbs of Akhkhyla (Abkhazian spice mix), and salt. Mix thoroughly Gradually add boiled, cooled water until the mixture has a smooth consistency. The mixture should look like the picture below.

Serving: Serve cold with chicken or turkey. We added walnut oil.

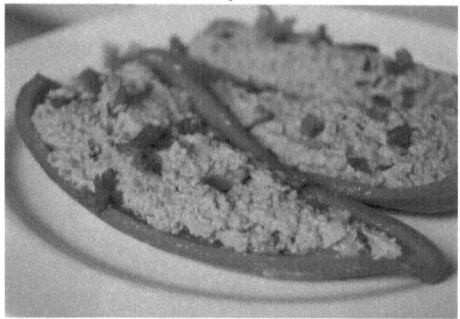

Apyrpylchapa is a dish from Abkhazia region made with marinated sweet peppers, walnuts and herbs. *Similar versions* are made in other regions of Georgia, especially in western Georgia.

Ingredients for filling: 6 large, sweet red peppers, 200 grams of walnuts, 1 tbs Ajika (click *here* for a recipe), 2 cloves of garlic, 1 onion, 10 grams of fresh parsley, 1 tbs of dried hot red pepper, 3-4 tbs of white wine vinegar, 50 ml of water, 10 grams of fresh green coriander, and salt (amount dependent upon personal preference).

Ingredients for marinade: 2 tbs of oil, 5 tbs of white wine vinegar (or pomegranate juice), 200 ml of water, 1 bay leaf, 1 tsp of sugar, 1 level tsp of dried hot red pepper, 1 clove of garlic, and 1 tsp of salt.

Preparation (marinade): Thinly slice 1 clove of garlic and add to a pan, together with 1 bay leaf, 1 level tsp of dried hot red pepper, 1 tsp of sugar, and 1 tsp of salt.

Add 2 tbs of oil, 5 tbs of white wine vinegar (or pomegranate juice) and 200 ml of water. Bring to the boil.

Slice the peppers in half and remove the seeds. Add to a bowl.

Pour on the marinade and leave for 30 minutes.

Preparation (filling): Finely chop the fresh green coriander and parsley and add to a mortar, together with 2 cloves of garlic. Crush and pound the herbs and garlic.

Grind the walnuts and chop the onion. Add to a bowl, together with the crushed coriander/parsley/garlic, 1 tbs of dried hot red pepper, 1 tbs of ajika, and salt (amount dependent upon personal preference). Add 3-4 tbs of white wine vinegar, and 50 ml of water and mix thoroughly.

Once the red peppers have marinated for sufficient time (at least 30 minutes), spread the filling on each slice of pepper.

Serving: Serve cold. We garnished ours with a little parsley.

C) Vilcabamba Recipes

No recipes are included from Vilcabamba in this edition of the book because all of my research led to modern recipes--not traditional ones. Still searching.

D) Hunza Recipes/Food Prep Guidelines

General Hunza cooking guidelines: (Classic, 1989)

1. Any kind of grains can be cooked and eaten with added oils, spices and sweeteners such as honey, maple syrup or fruit. Technically, when you make Hunza Bread, you are using grain. Another idea for the Dough is to spread it on a large sheet and roll it as thinly as possible (like a very large pancake). You can add any

toppings (more Veggies and Greens, and especially fresh garlic) that you like and what you end up with is a kind of Hunza Pizza!

2. Any kind of beans can be cooked. You can alter the tastes of any bean by adding flavorings such as onion, garlic, spices, oils, juices etc.

3. Soup is probably the most desirable COOKED food. Vegetable broths

are often much more potent suppliers of vitamins and minerals than the vegetable itself (and almost never cause indigestion, even in the most sensitive stomachs). You can make broths from any individual or combination of vegetables and ingredients. And, remember; when you are cooking vegetables

DON'T THROW OUT THE WATER! Drink it down. It, in fact, is just the broth that you'd make soup from and has all the vitamins that you've just cooked away.   When you make soups, blend your desired vegetables in a blender or chop them to your preference. Add natural herbs (go light on the salt) and SIMMER over a low heat. Make sure the cooking pot is covered and don't let the water boil the vegetables for too long (in fact, a steamer is preferable). Add spices if you like and eat the soup UNSTRAINED.   NOTE: Never fry or broil and never use oils when cooking.

A Recipe for Hunza Bread:

Hunza Diet Bread is a delicious, dense, chewy bread that's very nutritious and almost impervious to spoilage.

Hunza Diet Bread is made from natural buckwheat or millet flour, and is rich in phosphorous, potassium, iron, calcium, manganese, and other minerals. As nothing has been destroyed in the preparation from the wheat, it contains the essential nourishment of the grain. This is why it is important to **ONLY use Natural Buckwheat or Millet flour** to make Hunza Diet Bread.

The following recipe makes a huge batch of approximately 60 (sixty) two-inch squares, high in protein, vitamins, and minerals. It keeps weeks at room temperature, even longer in the fridge, and indefinitely in the freezer. It's a great survival food to take camping and hiking.

The recipe for this wonderful bread is as follows:

4 cups of water

3.5 (three & one-half) to 4 pounds of buckwheat or millet flour

1.5 (one & one-half) cups of coconut oil or canola oil

1.5 (one & one-half) cups of natural unrefined sugar

16 ounces of honey

16 ounces of molasses

4 ounces of powdered whey or soya milk (one-half cup)

1 teaspoon sea salt

1 teaspoon cinnamon

1 teaspoon ground nutmeg

2 teaspoons baking powder (non-aluminium)

While Hunza Diet Bread has a taste that is very satisfying and chewy all on its own, apricots, raisins, chopped walnuts, almonds, or sliced dates can also be added.

Mix all the ingredients. Grease and lightly flour your cooking pan(s).

Ideally, use baking trays with 1-inch-high sides.

Pour batter into pan(s) to a level of one-half an inch deep.

Bake at about 300 degrees Farenheit (150 C) for 1 hour.

After baking, dry the bread in the oven for two hours at a very low heat - 90 degrees Fahrenheit (50 C).

After the bread has cooled, remove it from the baking pan and cut into approximately 2 inch x 2 inch squares.

Store it wrapped in cloth in a container.

Fresh Fruit Ice Cream: (Classic, 1989)

In the form of ICE CREAM fruits can supply you with your nutritional needs AND satisfy the child in all of us. This method of utilization is also a sure favorite with REAL children. To accomplish this special recipe, place a combination of your favorite FRESH fruits into your freezer for 12 to 24 hours. When they are good and frozen, grind the mixed, frozen fruits through a meat grinder or other grinding machine. The results are largely a result of trial and error, depending upon the right combination of fruits to suit your tastes. What you'll get is an ice-cream-like substance without the cream or calories. You can add honey for extra sweetness, or carob powder and any other natural toppings that you prefer.

The Hunza Method Bread:

Blend the flour with salt (1/2 tsp. of salt for every two cups of flour) and add enough water to knead it on a lightly floured surface to prevent sticking. Knead until you have a very stiff consistency of dough, cover it with a wet cloth and leave it at room temperature for about one or two hours. At the end of that time, take the dough and shape small round balls (about 1 1/2 to 2 inches in diameter) and roll them on a lightly floured surface until you have a stack of pancake-like breads, about 10 to 12 inches across.

For natural yeast, keep one of the balls of dough under the wet cloth for 24 hours and mix it with your next day's batch of dough.

Cooking: The best method for cooking is to form the pancake like bread and NOT COOK IT AT ALL. Simply leave your formed cakes out in the sun, or in an oven with a temperature of UNDER 130 degrees. Another method is to leave the oven set low and THE DOOR OPEN. This will prevent the bread from cooking too fast, which destroys the nutritional value of the living grains. If you feel you MUST cook then, the second best method is to follow the recipe above and the procedures suggested, and then cook at a normal baking temperature.

Making Sprout 'Bread':

Here's a neat trick, you can also grind sprouts and knead the paste into stiff dough! Adjust the thickness of the dough, by adding small amounts of 100% stone ground whole wheat (or your favorite) flour, and small amounts of water. A little water makes your dough thinner, and a little flour does the opposite. When you get the consistency you desire, the dough can be used in the same way as was explained for bread and cake. As with breads and cakes, your own imagination is your only limitation in preparing the sprout-dough in a variety of shapes, sizes and recipes.

Diets and Lifestyles of the Worlds Oldest Peoples

Summary

This book is intended as a starting point for improving your health by losing weight and starting to live a healthier lifestyle.

We can best learn from what has worked for others.

The four communities in this book are historical labs which have experiential information on what long lived people actually eat and how they live.

The Diet Steps are just some guidelines to get your started. If you are serious about your optimal health then you should follow the path to take our longevity training too.

The Recipes which are included are designed to show you ways to prepare food as these longevity communities do.

My best wishes to you in improving and taking control of your life.

All the Best,

Marty Ettington

June 2015

Diets and Lifestyles of the Worlds Oldest Peoples

Bibliography

Alakbarli, Dr. Farid. Nutrition for Longevity. *azer.com*. [Online] [Cited: 5
31, 2015.]
http://www.azer.com/aiweb/categories/magazine/83_folder/83_articles/83
_longevity.html.

Davies, Dr. David. 1975. *Centenarians of the Andes*. s.l. : Barrie &
Jenkins, 1975.

2/1/2023. https://lyma.life/journal/how-to-increase-longevity-hunza-tribe-
secrets/. *How to Increase Longevity-Hubza Tribe Secrets*. [Online]
2/1/2023.

Okinawa Bridging Asia. Okinawa Bridging Asia. *http://www.jpn-
okinawa.com/*. [Online] [Cited: 6 6, 2015.] http://www.jpn-
okinawa.com/en/products/fruitsandvege/.

Robbins, John. Abkhazia: Ancients of the Caucasus.
http://abkhazworld.com/. [Online]
http://abkhazworld.com/aw/abkhazians/who-are-they/659-abkhazia-
ancients-of-the-caucasus.

Robinson, Paul Patrick. 2011. *An Operations Manual for Humankind*. s.l. :
Amazon Kindle, 2011.

Vilcabamba: the town of very old people. *Hoaxes.org*. [Online]
http://hoaxes.org/archive/permalink/vilcabamba_the_town_of_very_old_p
eople.

Wikipedia-Okinawa Diet Page. *Wikipedia*. [Online]
http://en.wikipedia.org/wiki/Okinawa_diet.

Wilson, Emily. 2001. *The Guardian.com*. [Online] 2001.
http://www.theguardian.com/education/2001/jun/07/medicalscience.health
andwellbeing.

Diets and Lifestyles of the Worlds Oldest Peoples

www.ingramcontent.com/pod-product-compliance
Lightning Source LLC
Chambersburg PA
CBHW050506290526
45786CB00006B/2453